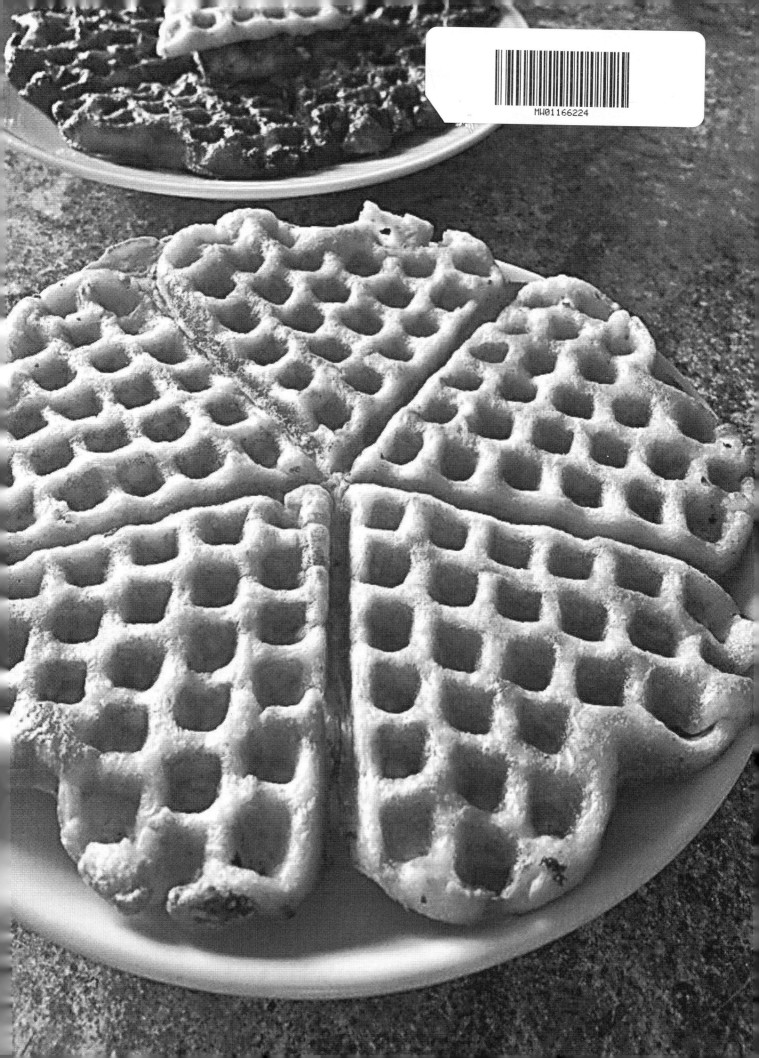

KETO CHAFFLE

RECIPES #2019

INCREDIBLE & IRRESISTIBLY LOW CARB KETOGENIC WAFFLES TO LOSE

WEIGHT, BOOST METABOLISM AND LIVE HEALTHY

Teresa Baker

KETO CHAFFLE RECIPES

INCLUDES RECIPE INDEX, NUTRITIONAL FACTS, AND SCORE POINTS GRADING

✓ EASE OF COOKING

✓ AVAILABILITY OF INGREDIENTS

✓ SPEED OF PREPARATION

✓ BUDGET FRIENDLY

✓ MEAL PREP FRIENDLY

✓ GROCERY EFFICIENT

✓ ALSO GLUTEN FREE, DIABETIC & PALEO FRIENDLY

BoldBar Publishing

Disclaimer

This publication is designed to provide competent and reliable information regarding the subject matter covered. However, it is sold with the understanding that the author is not engaged in rendering professional or nutritional advice. Laws and practices often vary from state to state and country to country and if medical or other expert assistance is required, the services of a professional should be sought. The author specifically disclaims any liability that is incurred from the use or application of the contents of this book.

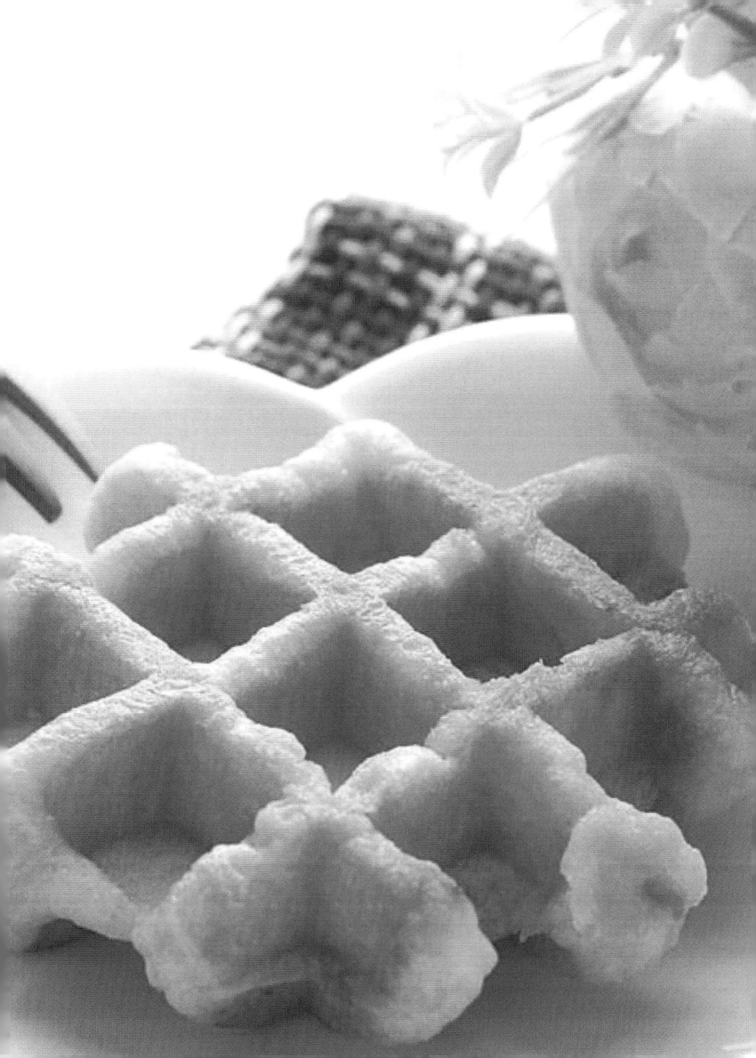

You May Also Like ...

Book Cover	Book Title	Purchase Link
	Keto Desserts Cookbook 2019 *Easy, Quick and Tasty High-Fat Low-Carb Ketogenic Treats to Try from No-bake Energy Bomblets to Sugar-Free Creamsicle Melts and beyond*	**Buy on Amazon**
	Keto Diet for Beginners 2020 *The Definitive Ketogenic Diet Guide to Kick-start High Level Fat burning, Weight Loss & Healthy Lifestyle in 2020 and Beyond.*	**Buy on Amazon**
	Keto Breakfast Cookbook *Simple No-Mess, No-Fuss Ketogenic Meals to Prepare, Boost Morning Metabolism and Ramp Up Your Energy!*	**Buy on Amazon**
	Keto After 50: *Keto for Seniors - 5g Net of Carbs, 30 minute meals	Lose Weight, Restore Bone Health and Fight Disease Forever*	Buy on Amazon
	Keto Lunch Cookbook *Easy Ketogenic Recipes for Work and School; Low Carb Meals to Prep, Grab and Go	With Q&A, Tips, and More..*	**Buy on Amazon**

Note that the Kindle Editions of these books will be made available to you for **FREE** when you get the paperback editions from the Amazon USA store

Contents

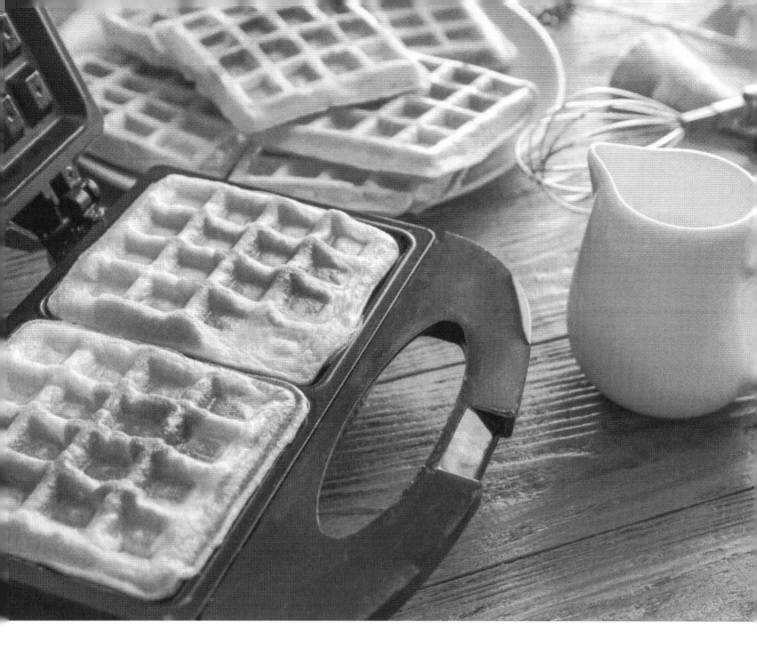

WHAT IS THIS BOOK ALL ABOUT?

This book contains steps and instructions, on how to start preparing healthy low carb Keto Chaffle meals especially if you want to lose weight fast, and live healthy. This book offers unique Keto Chaffle recipes that are completely sugar-free, gluten-free and healthy. In this book, you will also find several tips, tricks and strategies on how to get started and stay keto-adapted.

This Book features loads of keto Chaffles that you can tweak in many ways for a variety of flavors. Each recipe has a nutrient content guide per serving. Finally, it also contains a quick guide measurement conversion table that can come in handy when preparing your recipes. Prepare and enjoy these recipes while spending quality and enjoyable time with your family and friends. Teresa's tips also make it easy for anyone to get started and will guide you in ways to quickly achieve success on the Keto diet.

Without further ado, let's get started!

Specifically, in this cutting edge book, you'll discover Keto recipes that are:

- Quick, Easy and Simple to Prepare
- Under 5 minute chaffles
- Under 3g net of carbs
- Simple, precise, and defined preparation instructions
- Budget-friendly and very affordable
- Highly delicious and sugar-free wide range of recipes
- Gluten-Free, Diabetic and Paleo friendly
- Easily available ingredients

INTRODUCTION

Hello?

Finally, the cookbook you've been waiting for! The Keto Chaffle Recipe Cookbook!

This book will reveal the nitty-gritty secrets of the rave of the moment – Chaffles. How to make it - plus easy, delicious recipes anyone can prepare and much more!

The concept of Keto Chaffle is basically on the basic recipe – ½ cup cheddar cheese and 1 egg. So, basically,

Chaffles = Cheese + Waffles!

Enjoy the best compilation of the top mouthwatering Chaffle recipes. Without further delay, let's get started!

Basic Chaffle

Fluffy Keto Chaffle

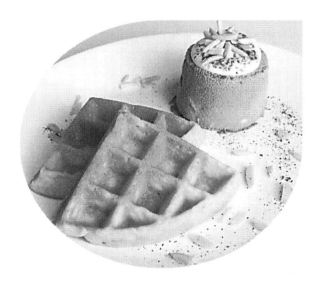

Prep Time: 3 min
Cook Time: 4 min
Total Time: 7 min
Servings: 1
Ingredients

- 1 egg
- 1/2 cup cheddar cheese, shredded

Instructions

1. Switch on the waffle maker according to manufacturer's instructions
2. Crack egg and combine with cheddar cheese in a small bowl
3. Place half batter on waffle maker and spread evenly.
4. Cook for 4 minutes or until as desired
5. Gently remove from waffle maker and set aside for 2 minutes so it cools down and become crispy
6. Repeat for remaining batter. Serve with desired toppings

Nutritional Facts (per serving):

- 291 calories
- 1g net carbs
- 23g fat
- 20g protein

Keto Sandwich Chaffle

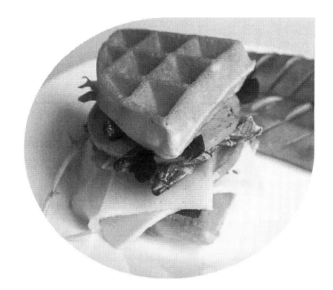

Prep Time: 3 min
Cook Time: 4 min
Total Time: 7 min
Servings: 1
Ingredients

- 1 egg
- 1/2 cup cheddar cheese, shredded
- 1 tbsp almond flour (optional)

Instructions

1. Using a mini waffle maker, preheat according to maker's instructions.
2. Combine egg and cheddar cheese in a mixing bowl. Stir thoroughly
3. Add Almond flour for added texture if so desired
4. Place half batter on waffle maker and spread evenly.
5. Cook for 4 minutes or until as desired
6. Gently remove from waffle maker and set aside for 2 minutes.
7. Repeat for remaining batter
8. Stuff 2 chaffles with desired garnishing to make a sandwich

Nutritional Facts (per serving):

- 170 calories
- 2g net carbs
- 14g fat
- 10g protein

Traditional Chaffle

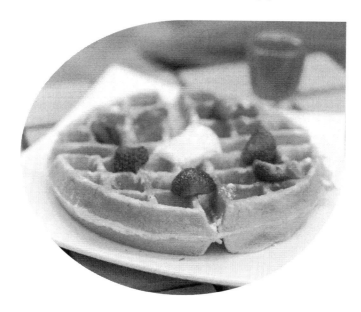

Prep Time: 5 min
Cook Time: 4 min
Total Time: 9 min
Servings: 2 mini waffles
Ingredients:
- 1 large egg
- 1/2 cup finely shredded mozzarella

Instructions
1. Switch on the mini waffle maker according to manufacturer's instructions
2. Spray the waffle iron with non-stick spray
3. Crack egg and combine with cheddar cheese in a small bowl
4. Place half batter on waffle maker and spread evenly.
5. Cook for 4 minutes or until as desired
6. Gently remove from waffle maker and set aside for 2 minutes so it cools down and become crispy Repeat with remaining batter.
7. Serve warm with desired toppings (optional) - butter, strawberries and sugar-free syrup

Nutritional Facts (per serving):
- 208 calories
- 2g net carbs
- 16g fat
- 11g protein

Fluffy Sandwich Breakfast Chaffle

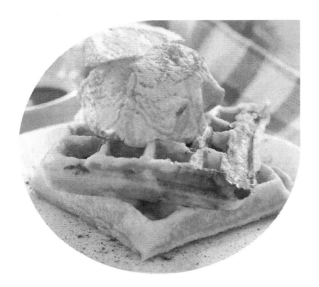

Prep Time: 5 min

Cook Time: 3 min

Total Time: 8 min *Servings:* 2

Ingredients:

- 1/2 tsp Psyllium husk powder (optional)
- 2 tbsp almond flour
- 1/4 tsp Baking powder (optional)
- 1 large Egg
- 1/2 cup Mozzarella cheese, shredded
- 1 tbsp vanilla or Dash of cinnamon

Instructions:

1. Switch on the waffle maker according to manufacturer's instructions
2. Crack egg and combine with cheddar cheese in a small bowl
3. Add remaining ingredients and combine thoroughly.
4. Place half batter on waffle maker and spread evenly.
5. Cook for 4 minutes or until as desired
6. Gently remove from waffle maker
7. Repeat for remaining batter. Top with keto ice cream

Nutritional Facts (per serving):

- 208 calories
- 2g net carbs
- 16g fat
- 11g protein

Keto Plain Prepped Chaffles

Prep Time: 3 min

Cook Time: 6 min

Total Time: 9 min

Servings: 2

Ingredients

- 2 small eggs
- 1/2 cup shredded cheddar cheese

Instructions

1. Preheat mini waffle maker until hot
2. Whisk egg in a bowl, add cheese, then mix well
3. Stir in the remaining ingredients (except toppings, if any).
4. Grease waffle maker and scoop 1/2 of the batter onto the waffle maker, spread across evenly
5. Cook until a bit browned and crispy, about 4 minutes.
6. Gently remove from waffle maker and let it cool
7. Repeat with remaining batter.
8. Store in the fridge for 3-5 days.

Nutritional Facts (per serving):

- 195 calories

- 1g net carbs

- 15g fat

- 14g protein

Vanilla Keto Chaffle

Prep Time: 3 min

Cook Time: 4 min

Total Time: 7 min

Servings: 1

Ingredients

- 1 egg

- 1/2 cup cheddar cheese, shredded

- 1/2 tsp vanilla extract

Instructions

1. Switch on the waffle maker according to manufacturer's instructions
2. Crack egg and combine with cheddar cheese in a small bowl
3. Add vanilla extract and combine thoroughly.
4. Place half batter on waffle maker and spread evenly.
5. Cook for 4 minutes or until as desired
6. Gently remove from waffle maker and set aside for 2 minutes so it cools down and become crispy
7. Repeat for remaining batter

Nutritional Facts (per serving):

- 291 calories

- 1g net carbs

- 23g fat

- 20g protein

Crispy Sandwich Chaffle

Prep Time: 3 min

Cook Time: 4 min

Total Time: 7 min

Servings: 1

Ingredients

- 1 egg

- 1/2 cup cheddar cheese, shredded

- 1 tbsp coconut flour

Instructions

1. Using a mini waffle maker, preheat according to maker's instructions.
2. Combine egg and cheddar cheese in a mixing bowl. Stir thoroughly
3. Add coconut flour for added texture if so desired
4. Place half batter on waffle and spread evenly.
5. Cook for 4 minutes or until as desired
6. Gently remove from waffle maker and set aside for 2 minutes so it cools down and become crispy
7. Repeat for remaining batter
8. Stuff 2 chaffles with desired garnishing to make a sandwich

Nutritional Facts (per serving):

- 170 calories

- 2g net carbs

- 14g fat

- 10g protein

Chia Keto Chaffle

Prep Time: 3 min

Cook Time: 4 min

Total Time: 7 min

Servings: 1

Ingredients

- 1 egg

- 1/2 cup cheddar cheese, shredded

- 1/2 tbsp Psyllium husk powder

- 1/2 tbsp chia seeds

Instructions

1. Switch on the waffle maker according to manufacturer's instructions
2. Crack egg and combine with cheddar cheese in a small bowl
3. Place half batter on waffle maker and spread evenly.
4. Sprinkle Chia on top and Cook for 4 minutes or until as desired
5. Gently remove from waffle maker and set aside for 2 minutes so it cools down and become crispy
6. Repeat for remaining batter
7. Serve with desired toppings

Nutritional Facts (per serving):

- 291 calories

- 1g net carbs

- 23g fat

- 20g protein

Keto Sandwich Chaffle

Prep Time: 3 min

Cook Time: 4 min

Total Time: 7 min

Servings: 1

Ingredients

- 1 egg

- 1/2 cup cheddar cheese, shredded

- 1 tbsp almond flour (optional)

Instructions

1. Using a mini waffle maker, preheat according to maker's instructions.
2. Combine egg and cheddar cheese in a mixing bowl. Stir thoroughly
3. Add Almond flour for added texture if so desired
4. Place half batter on waffle maker and spread evenly.
5. Cook for 4 minutes or until as desired
6. Gently remove from waffle maker and set aside for 2 minutes so it cools down and become crispy
7. Repeat for remaining batter
8. Stuff 2 chaffles with desired sandwich

Nutritional Facts (per serving):

- 170 calories

- 2g net carbs

- 14g fat

- 10g protein

Flaky Delight Chaffle

Prep Time: 3 min

Cook Time: 4 min

Total Time: 7 min

Servings: 1

Ingredients

- 1 egg

- 1/2 cup cheddar cheese, shredded

- 1/2 cup coconut flakes

Instructions

1. Switch on the waffle maker according to manufacturer's instructions
2. Crack egg and combine with cheddar cheese in a small bowl
3. Sprinkle coconut flakes and Cook for 4 minutes or until as desired
4. Place half batter on waffle maker and spread evenly.
5. Gently remove from waffle maker and set aside for 2 minutes so it cools down and become crispy
6. Repeat for remaining batter
7. Serve with desired toppings

Nutritional Facts (per serving):

- 291 calories

- 1g net carbs

- 23g fat

- 20g protein

Keto Minty Base Chaffle

Prep Time: 3 min

Cook Time: 4 min

Total Time: 7 min

Servings: 1

Ingredients

- 1 egg

- 1/2 cup cheddar cheese, shredded

- 1 tbsp mint extract (low carb)

Instructions

1. Using a mini waffle maker, preheat according to maker's instructions.
2. Combine egg and cheddar cheese in a mixing bowl. Stir thoroughly
3. Add mint extract and cook for 4 minutes or until as desired
4. Gently remove from waffle maker and set aside for 2 minutes so it cools down and become crispy
5. Repeat for remaining batter
6. Garnish with desired toppings

Nutritional Facts (per serving):

- 170 calories

- 2g net carbs

- 14g fat

- 10g protein

Spicy Chaffles

Garlic Bread Chaffle

Prep Time: 5 min
Cook Time: 4 min
Total Time: 9 min
Servings: 2
Ingredients:

- 1 clove Garlic, grated
- 1/2 tsp Italian seasoning
- 1/4 tsp Baking powder
- 1 large Egg
- 1/3 cup Parmesan cheese, grated
- 1/2 cup shredded Mozzarella cheese

Instructions:

1. Preheat mini waffle maker for about 5 minutes until hot
2. Add cheese and egg in a bowl and combine thoroughly. Stir in the remaining ingredients (except toppings).
3. Pour ½ of the batter into the waffle maker and spread well.
4. Cook until a bit browned and crispy, about 4 minutes.
5. Gently remove from waffle maker and set aside for 2 minutes so it cools down and become crispy
6. Repeat with remaining batter.
7. Top with extra melted cheese

Nutritional Facts (per serving):

- 182 calories
- 2g net carbs
- 11g fat
- 16g protein

Cinnamon 'Churro' Chaffle

Prep Time: 5 min
Cook Time: 4 min
Total Time: 9 min
Servings: 2
Ingredients:

- 3/4 tsp Cinnamon (for topping)
- 2 tbsp almond flour
- 1 large Egg
- 1/2 tbsp Butter, melted
- 1/2 tsp Cinnamon
- 1 tbsp Butter, melted (for topping)
- 3/4 cup Mozzarella cheese (shredded)
- 2 tbsp Erythritol
- 1/4 tsp Baking powder (optional)
- 1/2 tsp Vanilla extract
- 1 tbsp Psyllium husk powder

Instructions:

1. Preheat mini waffle maker for about 5 minutes until hot.
2. Add cheese and egg in a small bowl and combine thoroughly. Stir in the remaining ingredients (except toppings, if any).
3. Pour ½ of the batter into the waffle maker; spread evenly.
4. Cook until a bit browned and crispy, about 4 minutes.
5. Gently remove from waffle maker and set aside for 2 minutes so it cools down to become crispy.
6. Repeat with remaining batter.
7. Brush with melted butter and sprinkle with cinnamon "sugar" topping
8. Cut into churro sticks if so desired

Nutritional Facts (per serving):

- 179 calories
- 2g net carbs
- 14g fat
- 10g protein

Pumpkin Pie Chaffle

Prep Time: 5 min
Cook Time: 4 min
Total Time: 9 min
Servings: 2
Ingredients:

- 1/2 cup Mozzarella cheese (shredded)
- 1 large Egg
- 2 1/2 tbsp Erythritol
- 1/2 oz Cream cheese
- 3 tsp Coconut flour
- 2 tbsp Pumpkin puree
- 1/4 tsp Baking powder (optional)
- 1/2 tbsp Pumpkin pie spice
- 1/2 tsp Vanilla extract (optional)
- 2 tbsp Heavy whipping cream (topping)
- Dash of cinnamon (topping)

Instructions:

1. Preheat mini waffle maker until hot
2. Whisk egg in a bowl, add cheese, then mix well
3. Stir in the remaining ingredients (except toppings, if any).
4. Pour half of the batter onto the waffle maker, spread evenly
5. Cook until a bit browned and crispy, about 4 minutes.
6. Gently remove from waffle maker and let it cool
7. Repeat with remaining batter.
8. Top with whipped cream and cinnamon

Nutritional Facts (per serving):

- 117 calories
- 3g net carbs
- 7g fat
- 7g protein

Spicy Flavored Chaffle

Prep Time: 5 min

Cook Time: 4 min

Total Time: 9 min

Servings: 2

Ingredients:

- 1 cup Cheddar cheese (shredded)
- 1 large Egg
- 1 oz Cream cheese
- 2 tbsp Bacon bits
- 2 Jalapenos, sliced
- 1/4 tsp Baking powder (optional)

Instructions:

1. Preheat mini waffle maker until hot
2. Whisk egg in a bowl, add cheese, then mix well
3. Stir in the remaining ingredients (except toppings, if any).
4. Scoop 1/2 of the batter onto the waffle maker, spread across evenly
5. Cook 3-4 minutes, until done as desired (or crispy).
6. Gently remove from waffle maker and let it cool
7. Repeat with remaining batter.
8. Top with melted cheese, jalapeno slices, and bacon bits

Nutritional Facts (per serving):

- 231 calories

- 2g net carbs

- 18g fat

- 13g protein

Keto Seasoned Chaffle

Prep Time: 5 min

Cook Time: 4 min

Total Time: 9 min

Servings: 2

Ingredients:

- 1 large egg

- 1/2 c. shredded cheese

- Pinch of salt

- Seasoning to taste

Instructions:

1. Preheat mini waffle maker until hot
2. Whisk egg in a bowl, add cheese, then mix well
3. Stir in the remaining ingredients (except toppings, if any).
4. Scoop ½ of the batter onto the waffle maker, spread across evenly
5. Cook until a bit browned and crispy, about 4 minutes.
6. Gently remove from waffle maker and let it cool
7. Repeat with remaining batter.
8. Enjoy!

Nutritional Facts (per serving):

- 241 calories

- 2g net carbs

- 19g fat

- 12g protein

Keto Chaffle with Cream

Prep Time: 5 min

Cook Time: 4 min

Total Time: 9 min

Servings: 2

Ingredients:
- 1 large egg
- 1/2 cup shredded mozzarella
- 1 tbsp of almond flour
- 1 tsp vanilla
- 1 shake of cinnamon
- 1/2 tsp baking powder
- 1/2 tbsp whipped cream

Instructions:
1. Preheat mini waffle maker until hot
2. Whisk egg in a bowl, add cheese, then mix well
3. Stir in the remaining ingredients (except toppings, if any).
4. Scoop ½ of the batter on the waffle maker, spread across evenly
5. Cook until a bit browned and crispy, about 4 minutes.
6. Cook 3-4 minutes, until done as desired (or crispy).
7. Gently remove from waffle maker and let it cool
8. Repeat with remaining batter.
9. Top with whipped cream and cinnamon

Nutritional Facts (per serving):
- 271 calories
- 2g net carbs
- 27g fat
- 13g protein

Sweet & Spicy Chaffle

Prep Time: 5 min

Cook Time: 4 min

Total Time: 9 min

Servings: 2

Ingredients:
- 1 large egg
- 1/2 c. mozzarella
- 2 tbsp Stevia, liquid
- 1/2 tsp salt
- 1/2 tsp smoked paprika
- Pinch of cayenne pepper

Instructions:
1. Preheat mini waffle maker until hot
2. Whisk egg in a bowl, add cheese, then mix well
3. Stir in the remaining ingredients (except toppings, if any).
4. Scoop 1/2 of the batter onto the waffle maker, spread across evenly
5. Cook 3-4 minutes, until done as desired (or crispy).
6. Gently remove from waffle maker and let it cool
7. Repeat with remaining batter.
8. Top with whipped cream and cinnamon

Nutritional Facts (per serving):
- 252 calories
- 3g net carbs
- 21g fat
- 12g protein

Savory Herb Chaffle

Prep Time: 5 min

Cook Time: 4 min

Total Time: 9 min

Servings: 2

Ingredients:
- 1 large egg
- 1/4 c. shredded mozzarella
- 1/4 c. shredded parmesan
- 1/2 tbsp butter, melted
- 1 tsp herb blend seasoning
- 1/2 tsp salt

Instructions:
1. Preheat mini waffle maker until hot
2. Whisk egg in a bowl, add cheese, then mix well
3. Stir in the remaining ingredients (except toppings, if any).
4. Scoop 1/2 of the batter onto the waffle maker, spread across evenly
5. Cook until a bit browned and crispy, about 4 minutes.
6. Cook 3-4 minutes, until done as desired (or crispy).
7. Gently remove from waffle maker and let it cool
8. Repeat with remaining batter.
9. Serve and Enjoy!

Nutritional Facts (per serving):
- 294 calories
- 2g net carbs
- 24g fat
- 12g protein

Brownie Chaffles

Chocolatey Chaffle

Prep Time: 5 min

Cook Time: 4 min

Total Time: 9 min

Servings: 2

Ingredients:
- 1 large egg
- 1 oz. cream cheese, softened
- 1 tbsp ChocZero Chocolate Syrup
- 1/2 tsp vanilla
- 1 tbsp Stevia sweetener
- 1/2 tbsp cacao powder
- 1/4 tsp baking powder

Instructions:
1. Preheat mini waffle maker until hot
2. Whisk egg in a bowl, add cheese, then mix well
3. Stir in the remaining ingredients (except toppings, if any).
4. Scoop 1/2 of the batter onto the waffle maker, spread across evenly
5. Cook until a bit browned and crispy, about 4 minutes.
6. Gently remove from waffle maker and let it cool
7. Repeat with remaining batter.
8. Serve and Enjoy!

Nutritional Facts (per serving):
- 241 calories
- 2g net carbs
- 19g fat
- 13g protein

Keto Chocolate Chip Chaffle

Prep Time: 5 min
Cook Time: 8 min
Total Time: 13 min
Servings: 1

Ingredients

- 1 egg
- 1/4 tsp baking powder
- Pinch of salt
- 1 tbsp heavy whipping cream (topping)
- 1/2 tsp coconut flour
- 1 tbsp Chocolate Chips

Instructions

1. Preheat mini waffle maker until hot
2. Whisk egg in a bowl, add cheese, then mix well
3. Stir in the remaining ingredients (except toppings, if any).
4. Grease preheated waffle maker with. This will help to create a more crisp crust.
5. Scoop 1/2 of the batter onto the waffle maker, spread across evenly.
6. Sprinkle chocolate chips on top
7. Cook until a bit browned and crispy, about 4 minutes.
8. Gently remove from waffle maker and let it cool
9. Repeat with remaining batter.
10. Top with whipping cream
11. Serve and Enjoy!

Nutritional Facts (per serving):

- 146 calories
- 3g net carbs
- 10g fat
- 6g protein

Pumpkin Chocolate Chip Chaffles

Prep Time: 4 min

Cook Time: 12 min

Total Time: 16 min

Servings: 3

Ingredients

- 2 tbsp granulated swerve
- 1/4 tsp pumpkin pie spice
- 1 tbsp almond flour
- 1/2 cup shredded mozzarella cheese
- 4 tsp pumpkin puree
- 1 egg
- 4 tsp chocolate chips

Instructions

1. Preheat mini waffle maker until hot
2. Whisk egg in a bowl, add cheese, then mix well
3. Stir in the remaining ingredients (except toppings, if any).
4. Grease waffle maker and Scoop 1/2 of the batter onto the waffle maker, spread across evenly.
5. Add chocolate chips on top the batter and cook until a bit browned and crispy, about 4 minutes.
6. Gently remove from waffle maker and let it cool
7. Repeat with remaining batter.
8. Serve and Enjoy with some cream!

Nutritional Facts (per serving):

- 93 calories
- 1g net carbs
- 7g fat
- 7g protein

Mint Chocolate Chaffle

Prep Time: 5 min

Cook Time: 4 min

Total Time: 9 min

Servings: 2

Ingredients:

- 1 large egg
- 1 oz. cream cheese, softened
- 1 tbsp chocolate chips
- 1 tbsp Stevia sweetener
- 1 tbsp low carb mint extract
- 1/2 tbsp cacao powder
- 1/4 tsp baking powder

Instructions:

1. Preheat mini waffle maker until hot
2. Whisk egg in a bowl, add cheese, then mix well
3. Stir in the remaining ingredients (except toppings, if any).
4. Scoop 1/2 of the batter onto the waffle maker, spread across evenly
5. Cook until a bit browned and crispy, about 4 minutes.
6. Gently remove from waffle maker and let it cool
7. Repeat with remaining batter.
8. Serve and Enjoy!

Nutritional Facts (per serving):

- 241 calories

- 2g net carbs

- 19g fat

- 13g protein

Keto Coco-Chaffle

Prep Time: 5 min
Cook Time: 8 min
Total Time: 13 min
Servings: 1
Ingredients
1 egg
1/4 tsp baking powder
Pinch of salt
1 tbsp heavy whipping cream (topping)
1/2 tsp coconut flour
1 tbsp Chocolate Chips
Instructions

1.   Preheat mini waffle maker until hot
2.   Whisk egg in a bowl, add cheese, then mix well
3.   Stir in the remaining ingredients (except toppings, if any).
4.   Grease preheated waffle maker with non-stick cooking spray. Scoop 1/2 of the batter onto the waffle maker, spread across evenly.
5.   Sprinkle cocoa powder on top
6.   Cook until a bit browned and crispy, about 4 minutes.
7.   Gently remove from waffle maker and let it cool
8.   Repeat with remaining batter.
9.   Top with whipping cream
10. Serve and Enjoy!

Nutritional Facts (per serving):
- 146 calories
- 3g net carbs
- 10g fat
- 6g protein

Keto Vanilla Brownie Chaffle

Prep Time: 5 min

Cook Time: 4 min

Total Time: 9 min

Servings: 2

Ingredients:

- 1 large egg
- 1 oz. cream cheese, softened
- 1 tbsp ChocZero Chocolate Syrup
- 1/2 tsp vanilla
- 2 tbsp Stevia sweetener
- 2 tbsp cacao powder
- 1/4 tsp baking powder

Instructions:

1. Preheat mini waffle maker until hot
2. Whisk egg in a bowl, add cheese, then mix well
3. Stir in the remaining ingredients (except toppings, if any).
4. Scoop 1/2 of the batter onto the waffle maker, spread across evenly
5. Cook until a bit browned and crispy, about 4 minutes.
6. Gently remove from waffle maker and let it cool
7. Repeat with remaining batter.
10. Serve and Enjoy with topped melted butter!

Nutritional Facts (per serving):

- 241 calories

- 2g net carbs

- 19g fat

- 13g protein

Keto Crispy Choco Chaffle

Prep Time: 5 min

Cook Time: 8 min

Total Time: 13 min

Servings: 1

Ingredients

- 1 egg
- 1/4 tsp baking powder
- Pinch of salt
- 1 tbsp almond butter (topping)
- 1/2 tsp almond flour
- 1 tbsp Chocolate Chips
- 1 tsp cheddar cheese (reserve ½ for greasing)

Instructions

1. Preheat mini waffle maker until hot
2. Whisk egg in a bowl, add cheese, then mix well
3. Stir in the remaining ingredients (except toppings, if any).
4. Grease preheated waffle maker with 1 tsp of shredded cheese. Cook for 20 seconds. This will help to create a more crisp crust.
5. Scoop 1/2 of the batter onto the waffle maker, spread across evenly.
6. Sprinkle chocolate chips on top
7. Cook until a bit browned and crispy, about 4 minutes.
8. Gently remove from waffle maker and let it cool
9. Repeat with remaining batter.
10. Top with whipping cream
11. Serve and Enjoy!

Nutritional Facts (per serving):

- 146 calories
- 3g net carbs
- 10g fat
- 6g protein

Almond Chocolate Chaffle

Prep Time: 5 min

Cook Time: 4 min

Total Time: 9 min

Servings: 2

Ingredients:
- 1 large egg
- 1 oz. cream cheese, softened
- 1 tbsp ChocZero Chocolate Syrup
- 1/2 tsp vanilla
- 1 tbsp Stevia sweetener
- 1/2 tbsp cacao powder
- 1/4 tsp baking powder
- One handful almond nuts, cut in bit sizes (topping)

Instructions:
1. Preheat mini waffle maker until hot
2. Whisk egg in a bowl, add cheese, then mix well
3. Stir in the remaining ingredients (except toppings).
4. Scoop 1/2 of the batter onto the waffle maker, spread across evenly
5. Sprinkle Almond nuts, then cover and Cook until a bit browned and crispy, about 4 minutes.
6. Gently remove from waffle maker and let it cool
7. Repeat with remaining batter.
8. Serve and Enjoy!

Nutritional Facts (per serving):
- 241 calories
- 2g net carbs
- 19g fat
- 13g protein

Keto Chocolate Chip Chaffle

Prep Time: 5 min

Cook Time: 8 min

Total Time: 13 min

Servings: 1

Ingredients

- 1 egg
- 1/4 tsp baking powder
- Pinch of salt
- 1 tbsp cinnamon (topping)
- 1/2 tsp coconut flour
- 1 tbsp Chocolate Chips

Instructions

1. Preheat mini waffle maker until hot
2. Whisk egg in a bowl, add cheese, then mix well
3. Stir in the remaining ingredients (except toppings, if any).
4. Grease preheated waffle maker with. This will help to create a more crisp crust.
5. Scoop 1/2 of the batter onto the waffle maker, spread across evenly.
6. Sprinkle chocolate chips on top
7. Cook until a bit browned and crispy, about 4 minutes.
8. Gently remove from waffle maker and let it cool
9. Repeat with remaining batter.
10. Top with whipping cream
11. Serve and Enjoy!

Nutritional Facts (per serving):

- 146 calories
- 3g net carbs
- 10g fat
- 6g protein

Pizza Chaffles

Keto Pizza Chaffle

Prep Time: 5 min
Cook Time: 4 min
Total Time: 9 min
Servings: 2
Ingredients:

- 1 egg
- 1/2 cup mozzarella cheese, shredded
- Just a pinch of Italian seasoning
- 1 tbsp Pizza sauce (without added sugar)
- Shredded cheese, and pepperoni (or any favorite toppings)

Instructions:

1. Preheat mini waffle maker until hot
2. Whisk egg in a bowl, add cheese, then mix well
3. Stir in the remaining ingredients (except toppings, if any).
4. Add a bit of shredded cheese to the preheated waffle maker. Let it cook for 20 seconds. This will help to create a more crisp crust.
5. Scoop 1/2 of the batter onto the waffle maker, spread across evenly
6. Cook until a bit browned and crispy, about 4 minutes.
7. Gently remove from waffle maker and let it cool
8. Repeat with remaining batter.
9. Top with pizza sauce, shredded cheese, and pepperoni. Microwave on high for 20 seconds
10. Serve and Enjoy!

Nutritional Facts (per serving):

- 219 calories
- 2g net carbs
- 22g fat
- 12g protein

Delicious Pizza Chaffle Recipe

Prep Time: 5 min
Cook Time: 15 min
Total Time: 20 min
Servings: 2
Ingredients

- 1 egg white
- Pinch of salt
- 1 tsp cream cheese, softened
- 1 tbsp parmesan cheese, shredded
- 1/8 tsp garlic powder
- 1/2 cup mozzarella cheese, shredded
- 1/4 tsp basil seasoning
- 1/2 cup mozzarella cheese
- 6 pepperonis cut in half
- 1/8 tsp Italian seasoning
- 3 tsp low carb marinara sauce
- 1/4 tsp baking powder
- 1 tsp coconut flour

Instructions

1. Preheat waffle maker until hot
2. Whisk egg in a bowl, add cheese, then mix well
3. Stir in the remaining ingredients (except toppings, if any).
4. Add a bit of cheese to the preheated waffle maker. This will help to create a more crisp crust.
5. Scoop 1/2 of the batter onto the waffle maker, spread across evenly
6. Top with pepperoni, tomato sauce, and mozzarella and parmesan cheese. Microwave on high for 20 seconds
7. Cook 3-4 minutes, until done as desired (or crispy).
8. Gently remove from waffle maker and let it cool
9. Repeat with remaining batter.
10. Serve and Enjoy!

Nutritional Facts (per serving):

- 241 calories
- 2g net carbs
- 18g fat
- 17g protein

Spicy Pizza Chaffle

Prep Time: 5 min
Cook Time: 4 min
Total Time: 9 min
Servings: 2
Ingredients:

- 1 egg
- 1/2 cup mozzarella cheese, shredded
- A pinch of low carb seasoning mix
- 1 tbsp Pizza sauce (without added sugar)
- ¼ tsp kosher salt
- 1/2 cup heavy whipping cream (for topping)
- Shredded cheese, and pepperoni (for toppings)
- 1/2 tbsp Jalapenos slices (for topping)

Instructions:

1. Preheat mini waffle maker until hot
2. Whisk egg in a bowl, add cheese, then mix well
3. Stir in the remaining ingredients (except toppings, if any).
4. Add a bit of shredded cheese to the preheated waffle maker. Let it cook for 20 seconds. This will help to create a more crisp crust.
5. Scoop 1/2 of the batter onto the waffle maker, spread across evenly
6. Cook until a bit browned and crispy, about 4 minutes.
7. Gently remove from waffle maker and let it cool
8. Repeat with remaining batter.
9. Top with pizza sauce, shredded cheese, jalapenos and pepperoni. Microwave on high for 20 seconds
10. Serve and Enjoy!

Nutritional Facts (per serving):

- 219 calories
- 2g net carbs
- 22g fat
- 12g protein

Cheezy Pizza Chaffle

Prep Time: 5 min
Cook Time: 15 min
Total Time: 20 min *Servings: 2*
Ingredients

- 1 egg white
- Pinch of salt
- 1 tsp cream cheese, softened
- 1 tbsp parmesan cheese, shredded
- 1/8 tsp garlic powder
- 1/2 cup mozzarella cheese, shredded
- 1/4 tsp basil seasoning
- 1/2 cup mozzarella cheese
- 6 pepperonis cut in half
- 1/8 tsp Italian seasoning
- 3 tsp low carb marinara sauce
- 1/4 tsp baking powder
- 1 tsp coconut flour

Instructions

1. Preheat waffle maker until hot
2. Whisk egg in a bowl, add cheese, then mix well
3. Stir in the remaining ingredients (except toppings, if any).
4. Add a bit of cheese to the preheated waffle maker. This will help to create a more crisp crust.
5. Scoop 1/2 of the batter onto the waffle maker, spread across evenly
6. Top with pepperoni, tomato sauce, and mozzarella and parmesan cheese. Microwave on high for 20 seconds
7. Cook 3-4 minutes, until done as desired (or crispy).
8. Gently remove from waffle maker and let it cool
9. Repeat with remaining batter.
10. Serve and Enjoy!

Nutritional Facts (per serving):

- 241 calories
- 2g net carbs
- 18g fat
- 17g protein

Low Carb Pizza Chaffle Cups

Prep Time: 5 min

Cook Time: 4 min

Total Time: 9 min

Servings: 2

Ingredients:
- 1 egg
- 1/2 cup mozzarella cheese, shredded
- Just a pinch of Italian seasoning
- 1 tbsp Pizza sauce (without added sugar)
- Shredded cheese, and pepperoni (or any favorite toppings)

Instructions:
1. Preheat mini waffle maker until hot
2. Whisk egg in a bowl, add cheese, then mix well
3. Stir in the remaining ingredients (except toppings, if any).
4. Add a bit of shredded cheese to the preheated waffle maker. Let it cook for 20 seconds. This will help to create a more crisp crust.
5. Scoop 1/2 of the batter onto the waffle maker, spread across evenly
6. Cook until a bit browned and crispy, about 4 minutes.
7. Gently remove from waffle maker and let it cool
8. Repeat with remaining batter.
9. Top with pizza sauce, shredded cheese, and pepperoni. Microwave on high for 20 seconds
10. Serve and Enjoy!

Nutritional Facts (per serving):
- 219 calories
- 2g net carbs
- 22g fat
- 12g protein

Crispy Pizza Chaffle

Prep Time: 5 min
Cook Time: 15 min
Total Time: 20 min
Servings: 2
Ingredients

- 1 egg white
- Pinch of salt
- 1 tsp cream cheese, softened
- 1/8 tsp garlic powder
- 1/2 cup mozzarella cheese, shredded
- 1/4 tsp basil seasoning
- 1/2 cup mozzarella cheese
- 4 pepperonis cut in half
- 1/4 tsp Italian seasoning
- 2 tsp low carb marinara sauce
- 1/4 tsp baking powder
- 1 tsp Psyllium husk powder (for added texture)

Instructions

1. Preheat waffle maker until hot
2. Whisk egg in a bowl, add cheese, then mix well
3. Stir in the remaining ingredients (except toppings, if any).
4. Add a bit of cheese to the preheated waffle maker. This will help to create a more crisp crust.
5. Scoop 1/2 of the batter onto the waffle maker, spread across evenly
6. Top with pepperoni, tomato sauce, and mozzarella and parmesan cheese. Microwave on high for 20 seconds
7. Cook 3-4 minutes, until done as desired (or crispy).
8. Gently remove from waffle maker and let it cool
9. Repeat with remaining batter.
10. Serve and Enjoy!

Nutritional Facts (per serving):

- 241 calories
- 2g net carbs
- 18g fat
- 17g protein

Sweet & Savory Chaffles

Maple Pumpkin Keto Chaffle

Prep Time: 5 min

Cook Time: 4 min

Total Time: 9 min

Servings: 2

Ingredients
- 3/4 tsp baking powder
- 2 eggs
- 4 tsp heavy whipping cream
- 1/2 cup mozzarella cheese, shredded
- 2 tsp Liquid Stevia
- Pinch of salt
- 3/4 tsp pumpkin pie spice
- 1 tsp coconut flour
- 2 tsp pumpkin puree (100% pumpkin)
- 1/2 tsp vanilla

Instructions
1. Preheat mini waffle maker until hot
2. Whisk egg in a bowl, add cheese, then mix well
3. Stir in the remaining ingredients (except toppings, if any).
4. Scoop 1/2 of the batter onto the waffle maker, spread across evenly
5. Cook 3-4 minutes, until done as desired (or crispy).
6. Gently remove from waffle maker and let it cool
7. Repeat with remaining batter.
8. Top with sugar-free maple syrup or keto ice cream.
9. Serve and Enjoy!

Nutritional Facts (per serving):
- 201 calories
- 2g net carbs
- 15g fat
- 12g protein

Keto Almond Blueberry Chaffle

Prep Time: 5 min
Cook Time: 5 min
Total Time: 10 min
Servings: 5 Chaffles
Ingredients

1 tsp baking powder

2 eggs

1 cup of mozzarella cheese

2 tablespoons almond flour

3 tablespoon blueberries

1 tsp cinnamon

2 tsp of Swerve

Instructions

1. Preheat mini waffle maker until hot
2. Whisk egg in a bowl, add cheese, then mix well
3. Stir in the remaining ingredients (except toppings, if any).
4. Grease the preheated waffle maker with non-stick cooking spray.
5. Scoop 1/2 of the batter onto the waffle maker, spread across evenly
6. Cook until a bit browned and crispy, about 4 minutes.
7. Cook 3-4 minutes, until done as desired (or crispy).
8. Gently remove from waffle maker and let it cool
9. Repeat with remaining batter.
10. Top with keto syrup
11. Serve and Enjoy!

Nutritional Facts (per serving):

- 116 calories
- 1g net carbs
- 8g fat
- 8g protein

Keto Breakfast Chaffle

Prep Time: 3 min

Cook Time: 6 min

Total Time: 9 min

Servings: 1

Ingredients
2 tablespoons butter
1 egg
1/2 cup Monterey Jack Cheese
1 tablespoon almond flour

Instructions
1. Preheat mini waffle maker until hot
2. Whisk egg in a bowl, add cheese, then mix well
3. Stir in the remaining ingredients (except toppings, if any).
4. Grease waffle maker and Scoop 1/2 of the batter onto the waffle maker, spread across evenly
5. Cook until a bit browned and crispy, about 4 minutes.
6. Gently remove from waffle maker and let it cool
7. Repeat with remaining batter.
8. Melt butter in a pan. Add chaffles to the pan and cook for 2 minutes on each side
9. Remove from the pan and let it cool.
10. Serve and Enjoy!

Nutritional Facts (per serving):
- 257 calories
- 1g net carbs
- 24g fat
- 11g protein

Sweet Cinnamon "Sugar" Chaffle

Prep Time: 5 min

Cook Time: 4 min

Total Time: 9 min

Servings: 2

Ingredients
1/2 teaspoon cinnamon (topping)
10 drops of liquid stevia
1 tablespoon almond flour
Two large eggs
A splash of vanilla
1/2 cup mozzarella cheese

Instructions
1. Preheat waffle maker until hot
2. Whisk egg in a bowl, add cheese, then mix well
3. Stir in the remaining ingredients (except toppings, if any).
4. Scoop 1/2 of the batter onto the waffle maker, spread across evenly
5. Cook 3-4 minutes, until done as desired (or crispy).
6. Gently remove from waffle maker and let it cool
7. Repeat with remaining batter.
8. Top with melted butter and sprinkle of cinnamon.
9. Serve and Enjoy!

Nutritional Facts (per serving):
- 221 calories
- 2g net carbs
- 17g fat
- 12g protein

Keto "Cinnamon Roll" Chaffles

Prep Time: 5 min *Cook Time:* 10 min *Total Time:* 15 min

Servings: 3 chaffles

Ingredients

Cinnamon Roll Chaffle Ingredients

1/2 cup mozzarella cheese

1/4 tsp baking powder

1 tsp Granulated Swerve

1 tablespoon almond flour

1 tsp cinnamon

1 egg

Cinnamon roll swirl Ingredients

2 tsp confectioners swerve

1 tbsp butter

1 tsp cinnamon

Keto Cinnamon Roll Glaze

2 tsp swerve confectioners

1/4 tsp vanilla extract

1 tablespoon cream cheese

1 tablespoon butter

Instructions

1. Preheat waffle maker until hot
2. Add Cinnamon roll chaffle ingredients in a bowl and combine well
3. In another small bowl, add the cinnamon roll swirl ingredients and stir well.
4. Microwave for 15 seconds and mix well.
5. Spray the waffle maker with non-stick spray and add 1/3 of the batter to your waffle maker. Swirl in 1/3 of the "cinnamon roll swirl ingredient" mixture on top of it.
6. Cook for 3-4 minutes. Repeat for remaining batter
7. In a small bowl, add "Keto cinnamon roll glaze ingredients", combine and microwave for 20 seconds.
8. Drizzle on top of chaffles

Nutritional Facts (per serving):

- 180 calories
- 1g net carbs
- 16g fat
- 7g protein

Sweet & Savory Milky Chaffle

Prep Time: 5 min

Cook Time: 4 min

Total Time: 9 min

Servings: 2

Ingredients

- 3/4 tsp baking powder
- 2 eggs
- 4 tsp heavy whipping cream
- 1/2 cup coconut milk
- 1/2 cup mozzarella cheese, shredded
- 10 drops Liquid Stevia
- 1 tsp coconut or almond flour
- 1/2 tsp vanilla

Instructions

1. Preheat mini waffle maker until hot
2. Whisk egg in a bowl, add cheese, then mix well
3. Stir in the remaining ingredients (except toppings, if any).
4. Scoop 1/2 of the batter onto the waffle maker, spread across evenly
5. Cook 3-4 minutes, until done as desired (or crispy).
6. Gently remove from waffle maker and let it cool
7. Repeat with remaining batter.
8. Top with coconut milk and whipping cream.
9. Serve and Enjoy!

Nutritional Facts (per serving):

- 231 calories
- 2g net carbs
- 21g fat
- 12g protein

Sweet Raspberry Chaffle

Prep Time: 5 min
Cook Time: 5 min
Total Time: 10 min
Servings: 5 Chaffles
Ingredients

1 tsp baking powder

2 eggs

1 cup of mozzarella cheese

2 tbsp almond flour

4 raspberries, chopped

1 tsp cinnamon

10 drops Stevia, liquid

Instructions

1. Preheat mini waffle maker until hot
2. Whisk egg in a bowl, add cheese, then mix well
3. Stir in the remaining ingredients (except toppings, if any).
4. Grease the preheated waffle maker with non-stick cooking spray.
5. Scoop 1/2 of the batter onto the waffle maker, spread across evenly
6. Cook until a bit browned and crispy, about 4 minutes.
7. Cook 3-4 minutes, until done as desired (or crispy).
8. Gently remove from waffle maker and let it cool
9. Repeat with remaining batter.
10. Top with keto syrup
11. Serve and Enjoy!

Nutritional Facts (per serving):

- 116 calories
- 1g net carbs
- 8g fat
- 8g protein

Savory & Crispy Breakfast Chaffle

Prep Time: 3 min

Cook Time: 6 min

Total Time: 9 min

Servings: 1

Ingredients
2 tablespoons butter
1 egg
1/2 cup Monterey Jack Cheese
1 tablespoon almond flour

Instructions
1. Preheat mini waffle maker until hot
2. Whisk egg in a bowl, add cheese, then mix well
3. Stir in the remaining ingredients (except toppings, if any).
4. Grease waffle maker and Scoop 1/2 of the batter onto the waffle maker, spread across evenly
5. Cook until a bit browned and crispy, about 4 minutes.
6. Gently remove from waffle maker and let it cool
7. Repeat with remaining batter.
8. Melt butter in a pan. Add chaffles to the pan and cook for 2 minutes on each side
9. Remove from the pan and let it cool.
10. Serve and Enjoy!

Nutritional Facts (per serving):
- 257 calories
- 1g net carbs
- 24g fat
- 11g protein

Cake Chaffles

Chocolate Chaffle Cake

Prep Time: 2 min *Cook Time:* 8 min *Total Time:* 10 min *Servings:* 2 Chaffle cakes

Ingredients

Chocolate Chaffle Cake Ingredients

2 tablespoons swerve granulated sweetener

1 tablespoon almond flour

2 tablespoons cocoa powder

1 tablespoon heavy whipping cream

1/4 tsp baking powder

1 egg

1/2 tsp vanilla extract

Cream Cheese Frosting

2 tablespoons cream cheese

1 tsp heavy cream

1/8 tsp vanilla extract

2 teaspoons swerve confectioners

Instructions

1. Preheat mini waffle maker until hot
2. In a small bowl, add and whisk the "chocolate chaffle cake ingredients" until well combined. Scoop 1/2 of the batter onto the waffle maker, spread across evenly
3. Cook 3-4 minutes, until done as desired (or crispy). Gently remove from waffle maker and let it cool. Repeat with remaining batter.

Making the Cream Cheese Frosting

4. In a small bowl add the cream cheese and microwave for 10 seconds to soften.
5. Add in the remaining "Cream Cheese Frosting" ingredients and mix until fluffy

Assembling Keto Chocolate Chaffle cake

6. Place each chaffle on a plate, spread with a layer of frosting
7. Serve or refrigerate

Nutritional Facts (per serving):

- 151 calories
- 2g net carbs
- 13g fat
- 6g protein

Strawberry Shortcake Chaffle

Prep Time: 4 min
Cook Time: 12 min
Total Time: 16 min
 Servings: 3 Chaffles
Ingredients
Strawberry topping Ingredients

3 fresh strawberries

1/2 tablespoon granulated swerve

Sweet Chaffle Ingredients

1 tablespoon granulated swerve

Keto Whipped Cream

1 tablespoon almond flour

1/2 cup mozzarella cheese

1/4 teaspoon vanilla extract

1 egg

Instructions

1. Preheat waffle maker until hot
2. Whisk egg in a bowl, add cheese, then mix well
3. In a small bowl, add the strawberries and swerve; mix until well-combined. Set aside.
4. In another bowl, add the "sweet chaffle ingredients" and mix thoroughly.
5. Pour 1/3 of the batter into your mini waffle maker and cook for 3-4 minutes.
6. Rove gently and set aside to cool
7. Repeat for remaining batter – all makes 3 chaffle cakes in total.
8. Assemble the Chaffle by topping with strawberries and whipped cream.
9. Serve and Enjoy!

Nutritional Facts (per serving):

- 112 calories
- 1g net carbs
- 8g fat
- 7g protein

Keto Chaffle Taco Shells

Prep Time: 5 min

Cook Time: 20 min

Total Time: 8 min

Servings: 5 taco shells

Ingredients
1 tablespoon almond flour
2 eggs
1/4 tsp taco seasoning
1 cup taco blend cheese

Instructions
1. Preheat mini waffle maker until hot
2. Add ingredients to a bowl and mix well
3. Grease waffle maker with cooking spray
4. Add 1-2 tablespoons batter at a time to the waffle maker.
5. Cook for about 4 minutes.
6. Gently remove from waffle maker and drape over the side of a bowl or pie pan. Repeat with remaining batter.
7. Remove from the pan and let it cool.
8. Fill taco shells with favorite toppings
9. Serve and enjoy!

Nutritional Facts (per serving):
- 113 calories
- 1g net carbs
- 9g fat
- 8g protein

Mini Keto Pizza Chaffle

Prep Time: 5 min
Cook Time: 10 min
Total Time: 8 min
Servings: 2 Mini Keto Pizzas

Ingredients

- 1/4 tsp basil
- 2 tablespoons mozzarella cheese
- 2 tablespoons low carb pasta sauce
- 1 tablespoons almond flour
- 1/4 tsp garlic powder
- 1 eggs
- 1/2 cup Shredded Mozzarella cheese
- 1/2 tsp baking powder

Instructions

1. Preheat mini waffle maker until hot
2. Add all ingredients except pasta sauce to a bowl and mix well
3. Grease waffle maker and put half of the batter onto the waffle maker, spread across evenly
4. Cook until completely cooked, about 4 minutes.
5. Gently remove from waffle maker and let it cool
6. Repeat with remaining batter.
7. Once they are cooked, place them on the baking lined sheet in toaster oven.
8. Top each pizza crust with 1 tbsp each of pasta sauce.
9. Sprinkle with 1 tbsp each of shredded mozzarella cheese.
10. Bake at 350 degrees for 5 minutes, until the cheese is a little melted.
11. Remove from oven and let it cool.
12. Serve and Enjoy!

Nutritional Facts (per serving):

- 195 calories
- 2g net carbs
- 14g fat
- 13g protein

Vanilla Chaffle Cake

Prep Time: 2 min

Cook Time: 8 min

Total Time: 10 min

Servings: 2 Chaffle cakes

Ingredients

Vanilla Chaffle Cake Ingredients

1 tablespoon heavy whipping cream

2 tablespoons swerve granulated sweetener

1/4 tsp baking powder

1 tablespoon coconut flour

1 tbsp vanilla extract

1 egg

Cream Cheese Frosting

1/8 tsp vanilla extract

1 tsp heavy cream

2 teaspoons swerve confectioners

2 tablespoons cream cheese

Instructions

1. Preheat mini waffle maker until hot
2. In a small bowl, add and whisk the "vanilla chaffle cake ingredients" until well combined. Scoop 1/2 of the batter onto the waffle maker, spread across evenly
3. Cook 3-4 minutes, until done as desired (or crispy). Gently remove from waffle maker and let it cool
4. Repeat with remaining batter.

Making the Cream Cheese Frosting

5. In a small bowl add the cream cheese and microwave for 10 seconds to soften.
6. Add in the remaining "Cream Cheese Frosting" ingredients and mix until fluffy

Assembling Vanilla Chaffle cake

7. Place each chaffle on a plate, spread with a layer of frosting
8. Serve or refrigerate

Nutritional Facts (per serving):

- 151 calories
- 2g net carbs
- 13g fat
- 6g protein

Blueberry Cake Chaffle

Prep Time: 4 min

Cook Time: 12 min

Total Time: 16 min

 Servings: 3 Chaffles

Ingredients

Blueberry topping Ingredients

1/2 tbsp swerve

3 fresh strawberries

Sweet Chaffle Ingredients

1 tablespoon almond flour

1/2 cup mozzarella cheese

1 egg

1 tablespoon granulated swerve

Keto Whipped Cream

1/4 teaspoon vanilla extract

Instructions

1. Preheat waffle maker until hot
2. Whisk egg in a bowl, add cheese, then mix well
3. In a small bowl, add the blueberries and swerve; mix until well-combined. Set aside.
4. In another bowl, add the "sweet chaffle ingredients" and mix thoroughly.
5. Pour 1/3 of the batter into your mini waffle maker and cook for 3-4 minutes.
6. Rove gently and set aside to cool
7. Repeat for remaining batter – all makes 3 chaffle cakes in total.
8. Assemble the Chaffle by topping with strawberries and whipped cream.
9. Serve and Enjoy!

Nutritional Facts (per serving):

-   112 calories
-   1g net carbs
-   8g fat
-   7g protein

Avocado Chaffle Cake

Prep Time: 2 min
Cook Time: 8 min
Total Time: 10 min
Servings: 2 Chocolate Chaffle cakes
Ingredients
Chocolate Chaffle Cake Ingredients
1/2 tsp vanilla extract

1 tablespoon almond flour

1 tablespoon heavy whipping cream

2 tablespoons swerve granulated sweetener

1 egg

2 tablespoons cocoa powder

1/4 tsp baking powder
Avocado Cream Frosting
Half Avocado, chopped

1/8 tsp vanilla extract

1 tsp almond butter

2 tsp swerve confectioners
Instructions
1. Preheat waffle maker until hot
2. In a small bowl, add and whisk the "chocolate chaffle cake ingredients" until well combined. Scoop 1/2 of the batter onto the waffle maker, spread across evenly
3. Cook 3-4 minutes, until done as desired (or crispy). Gently remove from waffle maker and let it cool
4. Repeat with remaining batter.

Making the Avocado Cream Frosting
5. In a small bowl add the cream cheese and microwave for 10 seconds to soften.
6. Add in the remaining "Cream Cheese Frosting" ingredients and mix until fluffy

Assembling Avocado Chaffle cake
7. Place each chaffle on a plate, spread with a layer of frosting
8. Serve or refrigerate

Nutritional Facts (per serving):
- 151 calories
- 2g net carbs
- 13g fat
- 6g protein

Nutty Cake Chaffle

Prep Time: 4 min
Cook Time: 12 min
Total Time: 16 min
 Servings: 3 Chaffles
Ingredients
Strawberry topping Ingredients
1/2 tablespoon granulated swerve
½ cup almonds, chopped
Sweet Chaffle Ingredients
Whipped Cream
1 egg
1 tablespoon granulated swerve
1/4 teaspoon vanilla extract
1 tablespoon almond flour
1/2 cup mozzarella cheese
Instructions

1. Preheat waffle maker until hot
2. Whisk egg in a bowl, add cheese, then mix well
3. In a small bowl, add the strawberries and swerve; mix until well-combined. Set aside.
4. In another bowl, add the "sweet chaffle ingredients" and mix thoroughly.
5. Pour 1/3 of the batter into your mini waffle maker and cook for 3-4 minutes.
6. Rove gently and set aside to cool
7. Repeat for remaining batter – all makes 3 chaffle cakes in total.
8. Assemble the Chaffle by topping with strawberries and whipped cream.
9. Serve and Enjoy!

Nutritional Facts (per serving):
- 112 calories
- 1g net carbs
- 8g fat
- 7g protein

Advanced Chaffles

Keto Strawberry Chaffle

Prep Time: 3 min
Cook Time: 4 min
Total Time: 7 min
Servings: 1
Ingredients

- 1 egg
- 1/2 cup cheddar cheese, shredded
- 1 Strawberry, chopped
- ½ tsp Stevia, powder

Instructions

1. Switch on the waffle maker according to manufacturer's instructions
2. Crack egg and combine with cheddar cheese in a small bowl
3. Add remaining ingredients and mix well
4. Place half batter on waffle maker and spread evenly.
5. Cook for 4 minutes or until as desired
6. Gently remove from waffle maker and set aside for 2 minutes so it cools down and become crispy
7. Repeat for remaining batter
8. Serve with desired toppings

Nutritional Facts (per serving):

- 301 calories
- 2g net carbs
- 23g fat
- 20g protein

Keto Crunchy Chaffle

Prep Time: 3 min
Cook Time: 4 min
Total Time: 7 min
Servings: 1
Ingredients

- 1 egg
- 1/2 cup cheddar cheese, shredded
- 1 tbsp coconut flakes (optional)

Instructions

1. Using a mini waffle maker, preheat according to maker's instructions.
2. Combine egg and cheddar cheese in a mixing bowl. Stir thoroughly
3. Add flakes for added crunchy texture
4. Place half batter on waffle maker and spread evenly.
5. Cook for 4 minutes or until as desired
6. Gently remove from waffle maker and set aside for 2 minutes so it cools down and become crispy
7. Repeat for remaining batter
8. Stuff 2 chaffles with desired sandwich

Nutritional Facts (per serving):

- 175 calories
- 2g net carbs
- 14g fat
- 10g protein

Minty Keto Chaffle

Prep Time: 5 min
Cook Time: 4 min
Total Time: 9 min
Servings: 2 mini waffles
Ingredients:

- 1 large egg
- 1/2 cup finely shredded mozzarella
- 4 mint leaves, chopped

Instructions

1. Switch on the waffle maker according to manufacturer's instructions
2. Spray the waffle iron with non-stick spray
3. Crack egg and combine with cheddar cheese in a small bowl
4. Add mint leaves and mix well
5. Place half batter on waffle maker and spread evenly.
6. Cook for 4 minutes or until as desired
7. Gently remove from waffle maker and set aside for 2 minutes so it cools down and become crispy
8. Repeat with remaining batter.
9. Serve warm with desired toppings (optional) - butter, strawberries and sugar-free syrup

Nutritional Facts (per serving):

- 228 calories
- 2g net carbs
- 16g fat
- 11g protein

Green Breakfast Chaffle

Prep Time: 5 min

Cook Time: 3 min

Total Time: 8 min

Servings: 2

Ingredients:

- 1 tsp Matcha powder
- 2 tbsp almond flour
- 1/4 tsp Baking powder (optional)
- 1 large Egg
- 1/2 cup Mozzarella cheese, shredded
- 1 tbsp vanilla or Dash of cinnamon

Instructions:

1. Switch on the waffle maker according to manufacturer's instructions
2. Crack egg and combine with cheddar cheese in a small bowl
3. Add remaining ingredients and combine thoroughly.
4. Place half batter on waffle maker and spread evenly.
5. Cook for 4 minutes or until as desired
6. Gently remove from waffle maker and set aside for 2 minutes so it cools down and become crispy.
7. Repeat for remaining batter.
8. Serve with desired topping

Nutritional Facts (per serving):

- 249 calories
- 2g net carbs
- 18g fat
- 12g protein

Keto Protein Paffles

Prep Time: 3 min

Cook Time: 6 min

Total Time: 9 min

Servings: 2

Ingredients

- 2 small eggs
- 1/2 cup shredded cheddar cheese
- 1 oz Pork rinds, grated

Instructions

1. Preheat mini waffle maker until hot
2. Whisk egg in a bowl, add cheese, then mix well
3. Stir in the pork rinds.
4. Grease waffle maker and Scoop 1/2 of the batter onto the waffle maker, spread across evenly
5. Cook until a bit browned and crispy, about 4 minutes.
6. Gently remove from waffle maker and let it cool
7. Repeat with remaining batter.
8. Store in the fridge for 3-5 days.

Nutritional Facts (per serving):

- 395 calories

- 2g net carbs

- 26g fat

- 28g protein

Tomato Keto Chaffle

Prep Time: 3 min

Cook Time: 4 min

Total Time: 7 min

Servings: 1

Ingredients

- 1 egg

- 1/2 cup cheddar cheese, shredded

- 1 tsp tomato puree

Instructions

1. Switch on the waffle maker according to manufacturer's instructions
2. Crack egg and combine with cheddar cheese in a small bowl
3. Add puree and combine thoroughly.
4. Place half batter on waffle maker and spread evenly.
5. Cook for 4 minutes or until as desired
6. Gently remove from waffle maker and set aside for 2 minutes so it cools down and become crispy
7. Repeat for remaining batter
8. Serve with bacon

Nutritional Facts (per serving):

- 319 calories

- 2g net carbs

- 14g fat

- 11g protein

Plain Crispy Chaffle

Prep Time: 3 min

Cook Time: 4 min

Total Time: 7 min

Servings: 1

Ingredients

- 1 egg

- 1/2 cup cheddar cheese, shredded

- 1 tbsp coconut flour

Instructions

1. Using a mini waffle maker, preheat according to maker's instructions.
2. Combine egg and cheddar cheese in a mixing bowl. Stir thoroughly
3. Add coconut flour for added texture if so desired
4. Place half batter on waffle maker and spread evenly.
5. Cook for 4 minutes or until as desired
6. Gently remove from waffle maker and set aside for 2 minutes so it cools down and become crispy
7. Repeat for remaining batter

Nutritional Facts (per serving):

- 170 calories

- 2g net carbs

- 14g fat

- 10g protein

Keto Flaxseed Chaffle

Prep Time: 3 min

Cook Time: 4 min

Total Time: 7 min

Servings: 1

Ingredients

- 1 egg
- 1/2 cup cheddar cheese, shredded
- 1/2 tbsp flax seeds
- ½ tsp cinnamon

Instructions

1. Switch on the waffle maker according to manufacturer's instructions
2. Crack egg and combine with cheddar cheese in a small bowl
3. Place half batter on waffle maker and spread evenly.
4. Cook for 4 minutes or until as desired
5. Gently remove from waffle maker and set aside for 2 minutes so it cools down and become crispy
6. Sprinkle each with Flaxseed and cinnamon on top
7. Repeat for remaining batter
8. Serve

Nutritional Facts (per serving):

- 291 calories

- 1g net carbs

- 23g fat

- 20g protein

Keto Sandwich Chaffle

Prep Time: 3 min

Cook Time: 4 min

Total Time: 7 min

Servings: 1

Ingredients

- 1 egg

- 1/2 cup cheddar cheese, shredded

- 1 tbsp chia seeds (optional)

Instructions

1. Using a mini waffle maker, preheat according to maker's instructions.
2. Combine egg and cheddar cheese in a mixing bowl. Stir thoroughly
3. Add chia seeds and combine well
4. Place half batter on waffle maker and spread evenly.
5. Cook for 4 minutes or until as desired
6. Gently remove from waffle maker and set aside for 2 minutes so it cools down and become crispy
7. Repeat for remaining batter
8. Serve

Nutritional Facts (per serving):

- 170 calories

- 2g net carbs

- 14g fat

- 10g protein

Green Delight Chaffle

Prep Time: 3 min

Cook Time: 4 min

Total Time: 7 min

Servings: 1

Ingredients

- 1 egg

- 1/2 cup cheddar cheese, shredded

- 1/4 cup kale, chopped

Instructions

1. Switch on the waffle maker according to manufacturer's instructions
2. Crack egg and combine with cheddar cheese in a small bowl
3. Add kale, mix and cook for 4 minutes or until as desired
4. Gently remove from waffle maker and set aside for 2 minutes so it cools down and become crispy
5. Repeat for remaining batter
6. Serve with desired toppings

Nutritional Facts (per serving):

- 291 calories

- 1g net carbs

- 23g fat

- 20g protein

Lemon Minty Chaffle

Prep Time: 3 min

Cook Time: 4 min

Total Time: 7 min

Servings: 1

Ingredients

- 1 egg
- 1/2 cup cheddar cheese, shredded
- 1 tsp peppermint extract
- ¼ tsp Lemon, squeezed

Instructions

1. Using a mini waffle maker, preheat according to maker's instructions.
2. Combine egg and cheddar cheese in a mixing bowl. Stir thoroughly
3. Add peppermint extract and combine well
4. Scoop half batter and spread evenly on waffle maker. Cook for 4 minutes.
5. Gently remove from waffle maker and set aside for 2 minutes so it cools down and become crispy
6. Repeat for remaining batter
7. Sprinkle with lemon. Serve immediately

Nutritional Facts (per serving):

- 187 calories

- 2g net carbs

- 14g fat

- 10g protein

Keto Bacon Chaffle

Prep Time: 3 min

Cook Time: 4 min

Total Time: 7 min

Servings: 1

Ingredients

- 1 egg

- 1/2 cup cheddar cheese, shredded

- 2 tbsp bacon bits

Instructions

1. Using a mini waffle maker, preheat according to maker's instructions.
2. Combine egg and cheddar cheese in a mixing bowl. Stir thoroughly
3. Scoop half batter on waffle maker and spread evenly.
4. Sprinkle bacon bits, cover and cook for 4 minutes
5. Gently remove from waffle maker and set aside for 2 minutes so it cools down and become crispy
6. Repeat for remaining batter
7. Serve and Enjoy!

Nutritional Facts (per serving):

- 198 calories

- 2g net carbs

- 17g fat

- 14g protein

Power Paffles

Prep Time: 3 min

Cook Time: 4 min

Total Time: 7 min

Servings: 1

Ingredients

- 1 egg
- 1/2 cup cheddar cheese, shredded
- 1 tbsp coconut flakes
- Handful pork rinds, grated

Instructions

1. Switch on the waffle maker according to manufacturer's instructions
2. Crack egg and combine with cheddar cheese in a small bowl
3. Add coconut flakes and pork rinds; combine well
4. Cook for 4 minutes or until as desired
5. Gently remove from waffle maker and set aside for 2 minutes so it cools down and become crispy
6. Repeat for remaining batter
7. Serve with desired toppings

Nutritional Facts (per serving):

- 391 calories

- 3g net carbs

- 38g fat

- 35g protein

Keto Oreo Sandwich Chaffle

Prep Time: 3 min

Cook Time: 4 min

Total Time: 7 min

Servings: 1

Ingredients

- 1 egg
- 1/2 cup cheddar cheese, shredded
- 1 tbsp psyllium husk powder extract
- 2 tsp cacao powder
- 1 cup heavy whipping cream (coconut cream for non-dairy option)
- 5 drops liquid Stevia

Instructions

1. Using a mini waffle maker, preheat according to maker's instructions.
2. Combine egg and cheddar cheese in a mixing bowl. Stir thoroughly
3. Add husk powder and cacao; combine well
4. Cook for 4 minutes or until as desired
5. Gently remove from waffle maker and set aside for 2 minutes so it cools down and become crispy
6. Repeat for remaining batter
7. Stuff heavy cream between two chaffles
8. Serve!

Nutritional Facts (per serving):

- 495 calories

- 2g net carbs

- 24g fat

- 12g protein

Made in the
USA
Lexington, KY